CANCER IS A FOUR-LETTER WORD:

A Pilgrimage into the Emotional, Sexual, and Spiritual Aspects of Prostate Cancer.

To Karen,

Thanks for bringing your healing to others. The Word dances in and through you.

Blessings,

Larry

CANCER IS A FOUR-LETTER WORD:

A Pilgrimage into the Emotional, Sexual, and Spiritual Aspects of Prostate Cancer.

LARRY KREPS

PHOTOGRAPHY BY MARTI KREPS

authorHOUSE®

AuthorHouse™
1663 Liberty Drive
Bloomington, IN 47403
www.authorhouse.com
Phone: 1-800-839-8640

First published by AuthorHouse 12/14/2009

ISBN: 978-1-4490-6128-9 (e)
ISBN: 978-1-4490-6127-2 (sc)
ISBN: 978-1-4490-6126-5 (hc)

Library of Congress Control Number: 2009913472

Printed in the United States of America
Bloomington, Indiana

This book is printed on acid-free paper.

Foreword And Acknowledgments

"**Y**ou were the one we would have voted, 'Least likely to write an x-rated book,'" said a few of my old high school buddies after they'd read the first draft of my experiences with prostate cancer. My vocation is parish ministry, and it was obvious to them even as adolescents that is what I would eventually do. But prostate cancer is a very intimate disease, affecting men's private areas in ways that they'd never dream of talking about openly.

I am grateful to the men and their partners who shared their very intimate stories with me as I explored my own journey with the emotional, spiritual, and sexual aspects of prostate cancer. As I felt my way through the darkness of depression, fumbled for new expressions of sexuality, and lost my way with God, these men and women were lifelines leading me into a new and whole life. Their names have been changed to honor their vulnerability in sharing.

I am grateful to God's movement in the lives of men and women in the medical community who have researched and practiced lifesaving and life-giving skills, particularly our family doctor Barry Webb.

I am grateful to the family, friends, and congregation members of John Wesley United Methodist Church, who surrounded me with so much love that I could trust being honest with them and myself about what the experience of prostate cancer has meant for me. One gift of my cancer is the deepening appreciation and love for my wife Marti, our three children, and their spouses.

I am grateful to God, who enjoys arguments, questions, and doubts. Through better or worse, we are in life and death together.

I am grateful to the many who read this material and offered wonderful suggestions to increase the depth, accuracy, and clarity. Betsa Marsh and Coleen Armstrong provided editorial help and great encouragement. They pointed out things I should have remembered from eighth grade English. And, like all school English papers, I am the one finally responsible for the completed work.

I am grateful to my wife Marti, who held my hand at all the right times. We were at The Glen Workshop in Santa Fe, New Mexico, where I offered my first soul-baring draft of the book for critique. Before dinner one evening, a woman in my group came up and exclaimed, "I loved your writing. Thanks for sharing so personally."

I introduced her to Marti, and the woman turned red and was temporarily rendered speechless. Then she recovered. "I guess I know more about you," she laughed, "than you may want me to know!"

I am grateful Marti shares this vulnerable journey with me.

Markers for the Journey

This book can be read in a short time, or by pausing to consider and discuss the questions at the end of each chapter. The questions can prompt helpful conversation with a partner or support group.

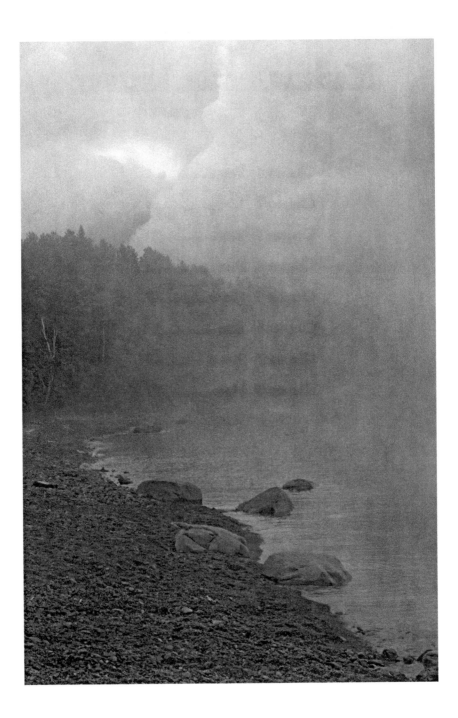

CHAPTER 1

FEAR

Twenty-five years ago I visited my grandfather in the hospital. Over the years I had listened to his stories of moving across France with the Marines and stopping the German advance at Belleau Woods, having a bomb drop into their campfire, and losing his hearing in one ear from a bullet. Now I sat beside his bed, waiting to hear whatever he chose to share before his upcoming surgery. He leaned his head back on the pillow and focused past the ceiling. Finally, he spoke: "The thing I feared most in World War I was having my balls shot off."

This statement came back to me this year as I recovered from the same surgery he'd had over two decades earlier. I am in my early fifties. He was in his early eighties. My cancer was detected early. His late. Mine was contained to the prostate. His escaped.

My life expectancy did not change. His life ended within a couple of years.

While grateful for my early diagnosis and treatment, I was surprised during my recovery by depression and a deep sense of loss. As I journaled one day, Grandpa's story came back to me, and with it the realization that cancer is not a six-letter word. It is four letters. Fear.

In September, 2006, I had my yearly routine physical. My PSA level, measured through a blood test, was not routine. The score was high compared to my baseline from two years earlier. PSA measures the prostate's response to anything foreign in its tissue, like infection or cancer.

I was referred to a urologist, and he signed me up for a biopsy and then handed me pamphlets on enlarged prostates and prostate cancer. I hoped for the enlarged prostate as cancer enlarged itself on my imagination. Cancer. The pamphlet said only ten percent of biopsies came back indicating cancer. So maybe being youngish for this disease, my odds were less than ten percent. But maybe my biopsy would come back clean, and I would think I was okay, yet in reality the cancer was present and undetected. Some days my fear stayed at ten percent; most days it soared higher.

The biopsy went smoothly. Then things got messy. The few days of antibiotic after the biopsy merely postponed the infection lingering in my system. A week and a half later, a urinary tract infection doubled me in pain. Urination and defecation were urgent yet nonexistent. A simple routine followed. Scurry to the bathroom, sit, groan, beat the wall with my hand, pass a bit, thank

God, and shuffle back to the recliner. Of course the infection hit on a weekend, making reaching doctors a challenge. Finally I got another prescription. Too late. Urination became nil. I squatted, stood, ran the faucets and showered, yet no urine flowed. At midnight on Monday I woke my wife Marti, groaning, "Sorry, but I need to go to the emergency room. I'm going to burst. Or not. Either way, I'm in trouble."

My wife and I have different recollections. She says they took us quickly, filled out the paperwork briskly, and had me in a room in short order. My memory is of the receptionist breaking off questions to get coffee, finish an e-mail to a distant cousin, and call home to confirm the shopping list for end-of-shift. Time is relative when agony is involved.

I did get to a room, and soon the pain of the infection and bladder gave way to the pain of the catheter insertion. I cringed and groaned through clinched jaw, but when the urine started running into the bag I gasped my thanks to the doctor and technicians. They grinned, holding up a full bag and said, "I guess you were in pain. This is as full as it gets."

The date was October 30. My birthday. The catheter, though not on my wish list, was the best gift ever.

Marti went with me for the appointment to hear the biopsy report. The doctor entered the room. "The biopsy consists of eight small tissue samples. You have cancer in three of the eight samples," he declared. "We think it is a mild, growing form and is not outside the prostate. Here is a brochure with treatment options. Read it, and I will be back in to talk about them."

Stunned, we struggled to focus on the brochure, reading terms like radiation seed implants, total prostatectomy, watchful waiting, and radiation.

I am a pastor. My attention skipped words on the page and landed on memories of being present with families when cancer was announced. The first time I ever waited with a family during surgery was as an intern in seminary thirty-five years ago. The doctor said the tumor had spread beyond what they could remove, and they could only close the incision and hope for the best. The family sat in numb silence, knowing the worst.

Announcements of breast, pancreatic, lung, and brain cancer to families over the years nearly always caused numbed silence, laced with fear. Questions followed. "How widespread is the cancer? Is this life-threatening? What treatments are available? What are the chances for survival?"

Many questions lurked unspoken beneath the spoken. "How will we tell our children? Will I be able to keep my employment? Should we spare telling our parent with dementia? How can this be happening?" All these questions became mine, battling for attention as I tried to read a brochure.

The doctor returned. He recommended books which outlined the nature of the disease and treatment options based on stage and age. He would see us in a week to answer questions and hear our decision. His calm did not mirror the increasing avalanche of our emotions.

SNAPSHOTS

William

William reported for physicals yearly, motivated by fear. His father had died an excruciating death from undetected prostate cancer. He made sure prostate screening through blood work and digital exam were included. When William's test came back positive for cancer, he acted quickly, doing research and choosing robotic surgery.

Charles

Charles' wife nagged him to get his PSA checked. Cancer had caused the death of his dad and many other male relatives. He figured cancer was part of his future, but not until his eighties, like his relatives. The results of his biopsy after a high PSA score surprised and shocked him. He was only in his mid-sixties. When Charles came home from the diagnosis, his wife immediately saw the news on his face. She ran and clutched him, moaning, "I don't want to lose you; I don't want to lose you."

Looking back, she now sees God's prompting in her "holy nagging." Charles is quick to point out that not all of her nagging is holy.

Harold

Harold heard his diagnosis at age forty-eight. By nature Harold is a rational, thoughtful person who sees a problem as something to solve. He approached the cancer as an illness which doctors could repair and his body as a machine that could be fixed. Choosing radical prostatectomy, the surgery revealed cancer spreading beyond the prostate.

Upon hearing the news, he thought of a baseball analogy. The original diagnosis was like the drama of pitching a tight game in the late innings. When he learned the cancer was already outside the prostate, it was like the leadoff hitter getting a single and then the next batter hitting a single and moving him to third with no outs. The situation called for urgency, focus, and determination. Harold had new problems to solve.

He began his radiation treatment with little fear, but more complications arose. The baseball analogy transformed into, "Cancer is more like playing with fire, a dangerous and unpredictable force."

DISCUSSION QUESTIONS

1. What were your first thoughts and feelings upon hearing your diagnosis?
2. Whom have you known who has had prostate cancer and what was their experience?
3. How is prostate cancer different from other cancers? Similar?
4. Where did you turn for help with your research on what treatment to select?
5. Do you tend to be a thinker or a feeler? How did this affect your actions and decisions?
6. What was the response by your partner or those closest to you?

Chapter 2

LOVE

Our first stop was the grocery store to refill a prescription for the urinary tract infection. As we milled around the pharmacy, our next-door neighbor saw us and asked if we knew the outcome of the biopsy. His wife is a breast cancer survivor. I opened my mouth, and the networking between my brain and vocal cords temporarily crashed. Several seconds later I whispered in staggered syllables, "I have cancer."

His tearing eyes held mine as he whispered back, "I'm so sorry."

We stopped next at church so I could tell our staff. This time tears filled the gap between what the brain wanted to say and the actual words. I said for the second time, "I have cancer."

Hugs of deep caring followed. As Marti and I drove down the street to our home I started to heave and cry. She pulled over and took my hand, and we sat. It was so hard to believe, so hard to know what was ahead, so hard to process.

The next hour I called our three children, my parents, sisters, and friends. Each time my voice caught on "cancer." Each time I knew I needed to say it, not only so the key people in my life would know, but also for me.

I continued this practice over the next few weeks. If someone asked how I was, I avoided the usual "Fine" and replied, "Not so good. I was just diagnosed with prostate cancer."

Conversations were then either short or long. I heard lots of stories of relatives and friends and special diets and cures beyond the mainstream. I did not mind. I was curious and hungry for information about this new world. Yet all this naming of "cancer" did not yet reach the depths of my knowing. This level of denial only became clear to me eight months later, after my successful treatment. Someone invited me to a banquet for cancer survivors. My first wonderments were, "Why are they asking me? Did they want me to pray for the meal?" No. I too was a cancer survivor.

One person I called the first night after diagnosis was Steve, whose prostate cancer had been surgically removed two years before. He buzzed right over on his motorcycle with his "Prostate Bible," Dr. Patrick Walsh's *Guide to Surviving Prostate Cancer*.

Steve speculated, "I imagine you are having all sorts of feelings. I sure was. The first thing I thought of was a friend who'd had a late diagnosis, and the cancer had spread beyond the prostate. Not good. Terrified, I felt in danger of losing my life and dreading what treatment might involve. Waking up in the night, with thoughts of the cancer dancing inside my head, I rose and sat in a chair to read more of Walsh. The book comforted me time and time again. I discovered that 92% of patients with my Gleason score of six had the cancer contained to the prostate upon surgery. That was a huge relief. I must have read that passage a dozen times!"

I got out the brochure the doctor had given me and looked at my notes. Mine was a six too. "The tumor could not be felt, and it is slow growing," I told Steve.

"You'll do great then," he said. "You are younger than I am and will heal better. I now look at it as a bump in the road instead of the end of the road. Did you know," he added, "a male can still have an orgasm even if he cannot have an erection or ejaculate?" My eyes got big, trying to comprehend a dimension of biology completely new to me. With a "Remember that!" he was off.

Through Walsh, I began to understand why something so small within my body could produce thoughts and emotions so large. I began to understand why my grandfather thought of having his balls shot off as he approached surgery.

The prostate is a walnut-sized gland that wraps around the male's urethra like a donut. It produces most of the semen that is ejaculated in intercourse. If the prostate enlarges due to cancer, infection, or aging, it grows outward and inward, the inward growth choking the urine flow. The constriction makes it difficult to empty the bladder completely, which is why many men begin to urinate more frequently in the middle of the night. Prior to 1981, doctors assumed the nerves controlling urination and erection ran through the prostate and had to be taken when the cancerous prostate was removed.

The side effects frighten many men, leading some to avoid physicals for detecting prostate cancer or avoiding treatment altogether. Patrick Walsh and Pieter Donker discovered the nerves could be spared, making the cure for prostate cancer much more bearable. The first question for many men after surgery now is, "Were the nerves spared?"

The words on the page were so clear and rational as I sat in my favorite recliner with my dog Alps. I'd read a paragraph or two, sigh deeply, set the book on my lap, and stroke Alps' head. I really enjoyed sex with my wife. I did not want to lose that very primal yet intimate part of love. I did not want to lose urination control. What would this do to hiking, jogging, basketball, and everyday activity? Reading some of the side effects of prostate cancer before the biopsy, I mused that if given the option, I would rather give up control of urination than sex. The urinary infection corrected my thinking. I pee much more often than I have sex. Later I heard one man say at this juncture that his doctor told him bluntly, "Dead men don't pee or have sex." Which nerves would be affected most and for how long? I laid my hands on my lower abdomen and prayed, "Dear Lord, bring your healing."

I felt no peace in this prayer, no confidence in my cancer disappearing. Against my theology of God's love for me, my prayer felt self-centered. Or was it that I did not trust God to bring healing? I knew God brought all kinds of healing. I had experienced in the lives of others healings that went against common medical knowledge. I also knew healing sometimes came nonphysically. I once asked a friend who led healing retreats for people with no further medical options for cancer, "Is everyone healed?"

"Yes," he said, "but in different ways. There were times the cancer disappeared, but most times healing took place within their spirit. They came to a peaceful acceptance of their disease, the awareness of the profound love of God in the midst of difficulty. Sometimes the retreat allowed people to be aware of broken relationships that needed tending in the shadow of their coming death. Often they found ways to reach out and mend, or let go of past hurts."

As I sat quietly with my awkwardness, I sensed my healing would not be supernatural. I would need to trust my cancer to God's activity--working through the knowledge and skill of the medical community.

Many people were praying for me. One friend knitted a prayer shawl. Each click of the knitting needles signaled a prayer for my well-being. As I sat with Alps and my journal in the morning chill of late fall, I draped that shawl around me for warmth and comfort.

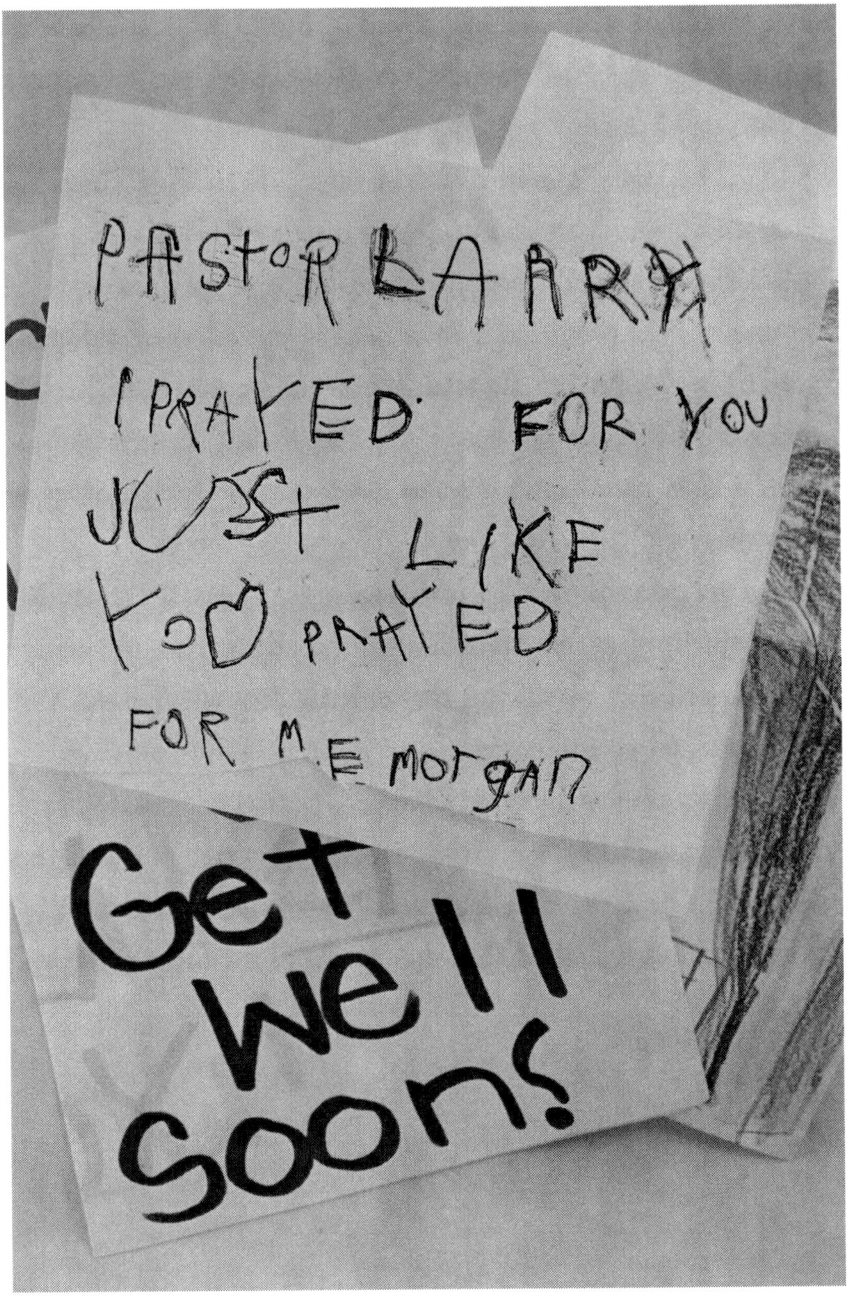
PASTOR BARRY
I PRAYED FOR YOU
JUST LIKE
YOU PRAYED
FOR ME morgan
Get
Well
Soon!

The children of the church wrote get-well cards. One four-year-old worked on hers for a week. Several years before as a baby on Christmas Eve, Morgan's parents rushed her to the children's hospital in a life-threatening situation. I spent the night with the family until Christmas dawn, when we received word that all would be well.

As I waited for my treatment, little Morgan and her grandmother walked up to me after church. Morgan, hiding behind her grandmother, extended her hand with a pasted, glittered card, "Dear Pastor Larry, You prayed for me. I am praying for you. Love, Morgan." I knelt, and she came to me. I hugged her as my tears touched her hair.

A phrase I used often when people asked how I was doing during these days was, "I feel carried by God's love and so many people's love." I was not at my best emotionally, physically, or spiritually, but I did not need to be. I was carried.

Some people assured me all would be well. They had a deep sense of peace about the outcome. Each looked me in the eye with compassion and spoke from deep within. I did not know what they meant exactly. Would I be cured of the cancer so no treatment would be necessary? Would the treatment go well? Would I come to a place of peaceful acceptance of whatever transpired? Later on, so moved by the quantity of heartfelt prayers offered on my behalf, I would go for one last PSA test to determine if I still had cancer before starting treatment.

When the results came back that the cancer was growing, I was surprised by my disappointment. I had still hoped for healing in a non-medical way. No miracle cure for me.

The next two months were a powerful mix of business, family, major church events, and anxious, watchful waiting. The strands were woven together so closely, each part touched the other. As a congregation, we moved through the pre-Christmas season to Christmas Eve. There was plenty to keep my mind occupied, but not so occupied that as I prepared my Christmas Eve sermon I didn't think, "What if this is my last Christmas to preach? What do I really want to say?"

I did not mention this to anyone on Christmas Eve, and no one came out of the service saying, "Wow! That was your best ever!" But I was very aware as I offered the sermon to God and the congregation.

Our extended family Christmas gatherings are large, since I have four sisters and sixteen nephews and nieces on one side. Several of the nephews and nieces who were in their twenties wrote me letters after the diagnosis with encouraging words and specific incidents from the past of about how much I meant to them. Seeing them face-to-face, I was near tears the entire afternoon. A couple of days after Christmas, my three children and their two spouses and fiancé joined us for our Christmas. We opened presents, and then sat down for our breakfast of bacon and waffles topped with ice cream. I looked around the table and started to weep. These were my most important people. I loved them. I needed them. I did not want to leave them. Gratitude mingled with fear of losing them. I could see the fragile threads that connected us, so precious and beautiful. I held the threads gently in my vision, wondering how long those threads would be unbroken. A year? Ten years? Thirty?

One special Christmas gift came from a friend surviving breast cancer. It had been given to her as she approached surgery. I opened the wrapping to discover a journal. The card explained, "A friend gave me a journal when I was ill and really encouraged me to put down three things a day that I was grateful for. I found it very helpful––it shifted my thinking on even the bleakest days. Gratitude is a good thing to cultivate."

Each night I turned off the living room light, settled on the couch, and opened the journal in the light of the Christmas tree and wrote:

o   The familiarity of Marti's hand and the warmth that spreads within me as we touch.
o   Alps nestling beside me in the chair when I read.
o   The gift of medical insurance.
o   Watching my son's face go from casual interest to fear to determination in selecting an engagement ring.
o   My daughter coming home and giving me a big hug and her energy.
o   A full moon in the early evening sky.
o   The ability to feel emotions, even anger, sadness, and disappointment.

My Gratitude Journal did not take away the fears of loss of urination, erection, or even life, but night after night it became an oasis of contentedness. I was thankful for so much. The anticipation of needing to list gratitudes that evening kept me alert all day to blessings. Rarely did I limit an entry to three. I became more likely to say thanks to people during the day.

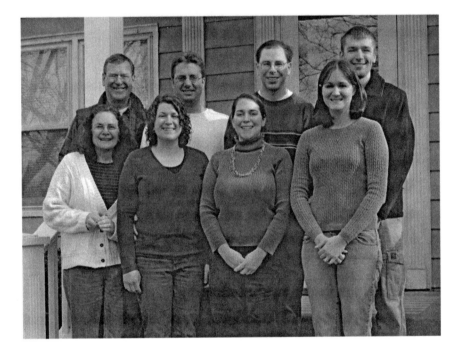

SNAPSHOTS

Harold

This question led to a pause in Harold's analytical thinking: "When did you feel God's love in your diagnosis, treatments, and recovery?" Not one for emotion, his own tear forming on the side of his eye surprised him. "There were a couple of times, no, three. One was being whisked away on a gurney to surgery. I went through a mental checklist. Bills paid? Check. Bank statement balanced? Check. Things wrapped up at work? Check. I realized I had done all I could do and whispered, 'God, I'm in your hands.' An amazing peace came." He paused, as if he were back in that peace.

Shaking his head a bit, he continued, "And when I needed follow up treatment at a distant hospital, my son flew in to drive my wife and me. The only comfortable position for me was curled up on the back seat. As he drove, I felt his love, like when I used to drive him places as a boy, and glance at him in the back seat just to see him."

After another pause, I asked, "And the third?"

"Well, actually four. The third was one night when some church friends stopped at the house, people who had kept track of me through this. I was eight years out from surgery and radiation, and having trouble with all kinds of internal scarring and undetermined infections. They came by to encourage me to go out of town for an evaluation. I was deeply touched by their caring. I did go, and finally found some relief at an excellent regional hospital."

Before I could say, "Fourth?" he said, "And my wife. She knows me, that I struggle with expressing or even acknowledging that I have feelings. She found ways to express her worry to others and to be a rock for me. She went to all of my doctor appointments and treatments."

The tears actually came as he softly said, "She has been wonderful."

DISCUSSION QUESTIONS

1. With whom did you choose to share your news and why?

2. How did you share the news about your cancer to family, friends, neighbors, and work associates?

3. What was it like to share this news?

4. What specific acts of tenderness have meant a lot to you?

5. What actions by family and friends meant a great deal to you?

6. When have you felt close as a couple during diagnosis, treatment, and recovery?

7. What have been the most frustrating times?

CHAPTER 3

PICK

Trying to determine which kind of treatment to pursue was daunting. A prostate cancer patient is given so many choices because there are several valid options with differing inputs and outcomes. Some men want to do whatever it takes to eradicate the cancer as soon as possible. Some need immediate attention because the cancer is fast-growing or has already breached the prostate. Some choose active surveillance, a process of watching and waiting, hoping they will not have to seek treatment that might result in urinary or erection difficulties. A man in his eighties might well do nothing. Other diseases would most likely bring his death well before the prostate cancer would.

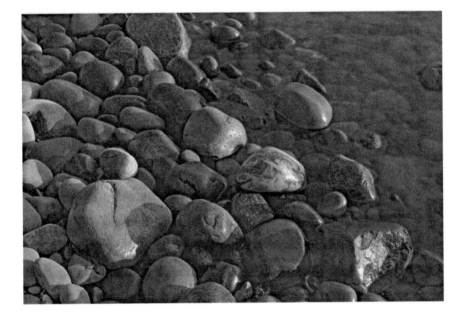

My cancer was grade 1, stage A, with a Gleason score of six. This meant that my cancer cells were most likely uniform, closely packed, and in the center of the prostate where they could not be felt. The tumor was mild-growing and contained within the prostate, where it could be totally removed. Doctors could not be certain, but the preliminary news was good.

I had time to consider which option would most likely eradicate the cancer. Being fifty-two, actually fifty-three on the date of the catheter gift, the main consideration was to use the method most likely to remove all of it, as I hoped for many years to live. This involved surgery. If the surgery did not work, other methods could be tried, like radiation. But if other methods were tried first and failed, surgery was not as good an option. In selecting a surgeon, "the prostate Bible" (<u>Dr. Patrick Walsh's Guide to Surviving Prostate Cancer, Second Edition</u>), delivered by Steve on his motorcycle, recommended choosing a surgeon who was well-experienced, with at least three hundred surgeries, still performing many each week.

But with surgery, how severe would the damage to the nerves controlling urination and erection be? I called several men who had been through the surgery. One said, "I had it six months ago, and I can have enough erection for a soft penetration. As healing goes on, it should become firmer."

Another echoed my motorcycle friend: "I still don't have an erection without the help of a pill, but the orgasm is still good."

One man declined to tell me his story until after my treatment. He was merciful. As he told me later, his recovery had involved complication after complication. He needed additional surgery for

25

urinary control and never was able to have erections, even with all of the treatments available for erectile dysfunction.

All of this, particularly the issues of incontinence and erectile dysfunction, were still outside my experience and comprehension. The books and pamphlets did not go into as much detail as the men shared with me. Hearing them gave me hope that even if there was erectile dysfunction, my wife and I could find ways for sexual expression.

Contacts came through friends, parishioners, and friends of parishioners. I called each one. Each story was a little different but brought reality and hope. One was a son of one of my mother's friends. Just months earlier, he'd had a new kind of surgery done, robotic. The robot, controlled by the surgeon, reportedly could see more clearly the surgery site because of greater magnification and less blood loss. The robot could also cut more precisely. The surgery was new to our area, but the surgeon at a large university hospital a hundred miles away had done as many as anyone in the world.

I checked on a variety of procedures through books and online resources, including external radiation, radiation seeds, proton beam therapy, traditional open surgery, and robotic. Any man I knew of having used these treatments I quizzed on the details and recovery. The Prostate Cancer Institute (1-866-469-7733) afforded me the opportunity to talk with a medical professional about my case.

I shared my research with my wife and a few of the men who had already had treatment. I leaned toward open or robotic surgery. My wife and I saw both the urologist and family doctor and shared with them a list of surgeons we planned to interview before making a final decision. They both concurred that these surgeons were good. We interviewed one locally and the one a hundred miles away. We chose distance over convenience. We signed up for robotic surgery for February 9, 2007.

The decision would be tested. I knew it would. As a public figure, I live in a glass bowl of sorts. I wondered how my research in books, conversations, doctors, and prayer would hold up after I announced my plans publicly. The congregation fulfilled my expectations. Most had never heard of robotic surgery and wondered if the procedure was too untested. They wondered why I was going out of town for treatment. Should I be taking so long to make my decision and be treated? My explanations sounded good to them, and as they did their own independent checking, they came back with their encouragement.

My peace persisted. It was now mid-November. Two months to go.

Usually our congregation worships at three different worship services. The Sunday before my surgery we consecrated a new multi-use space with one worship service. The building represented a culmination of many gifts of time and finances, and a new resource for ministry in the community. The morning of the service, greeters and ushers went about their responsibilities, but hid something whenever I glanced their way. I discovered what it was when, on cue during worship, everyone lifted his or her arm showing a blue *UsToo Prostate Cancer Education and Support Organization* wristband. My eyes filled with tears, one running from my eye to my chin.

The surgery was to take place on Friday, February 9, 2007. On the Wednesday before at staff meeting, they sat me in a chair and surrounded me. They chose two ancient acts to bless me. Placing hands on my shoulders and head, they offered prayers and anointed my forehead with oil. On the day of the surgery, several people would gather in the sanctuary to pray while it took place. I felt very loved.

Marti and I left on Thursday afternoon and spent the night with friends. Waking at five in the morning, Marti took a shower as I read a Scripture that I'd first read in high school while in the hospital for a short stay.

"Therefore I tell you, do not be anxious about your life, what you shall eat or what you shall drink, nor about your body, what you shall put on. Is not life more than food, and the body more than clothing? Look at the birds of the air; they neither sow nor reap nor gather into barns, and yet your heavenly Father feeds them. Are you not of more value than they? And which of you by being anxious can add one cubit to his span of life? Therefore do not be anxious. But seek first his kingdom and his righteousness, and all these things shall be yours as well. Therefore do not be anxious about tomorrow, for tomorrow will be anxious for itself. Let the day's own trouble be sufficient for the day." Matthew 6:25-27, 31, 34.

I read it again because I still felt anxious. Would pain be severe? Had the cancer spread beyond the prostate, sending poisonous cells through my tissue and organs? Did we just experience intercourse for the last time? How long would diapers and pads be needed to catch and soak up urine?

As I showered, I rewrote the Scripture in my head, hoping it would also be in my depths in the unknown days, weeks, months, and years ahead. "God, are You not more than cancer, more than urination, more than sex? You are my God through all generations and today. I will seek first Your kingdom and righteousness; all else will fall into place."

Cleansed by Scripture, prayer, shower, and an enema, I was as ready as I could be. Nervous, but anchored.

I chatted my way through the registration process, discovering that the young lady taking our information was a college student soon to be married. She was a United Methodist like me, and from a small church in northeast Ohio. The anesthesiologist shared that he too was a United Methodist, and taught fourth-grade Sunday school. He asked me, "How many of each animal did Moses take on the ark?"

My brain froze. Fortunately Marti jumped in with, "Zero. It was Noah and the ark."

My parents arrived. A friend came and prayed for us, and then I was wheeled away. We passed the robot room, and I asked if the robot had a nickname. The orderly did not know. Disappointed by my failed attempt at levity, I rolled toward my grandfather's and my fear of having our balls blown off. Temporarily pushed into a curtained area, I waited, breathing in God's Spirit, exhaling anxiety, keeping my hands on my lower abdomen for healing touch. The hour of healing was here. I awoke on the other side of surgery.

SNAPSHOTS

Hank

The news of Hank's cancer came toward the end of his wife's fifteen-year struggle with breast cancer. He opted for radiation seeds, since his recovery period would be shorter than other treatments. Hank wanted to be fully present to his wife in her struggles. He was. One year later she died under Hospice care.

Mike

Mike delayed any treatment for a year, as within days of his diagnosis, his wife fell. Her ensuing scans revealed a brain tumor that biopsy proved to be malignant. Mike stayed by her side for her final two months. Surgery for his prostate came a year later.

DISCUSSION QUESTIONS

1. What were the end results most important to you in choosing a treatment?
2. What procedures did you want to research and by what means?
3. Which doctors did you want to interview?
4. Make a chart or spreadsheet that can help you keep track of the pros and cons for each treatment.
5. With whom would you like to share your thinking before making a decision?

Chapter 4

PAIN

Pain medication is wonderful! I felt even better when I heard everything looked to be as expected with the cancer contained in the prostate. A biopsy would be done to make sure, but preliminary indications were good. Extremely large, the prostate attached to surrounding tissue, so it took more time to extricate. The robot handled the complication with ease.

I sat up late Friday afternoon, the day of surgery and healing. Marti and I strolled down the hall in the evening. Instead of Alps' pitter-patter at our feet, a mobile IV unit glided at my side.

The next morning the nurse explained care for the wound, the catheter, and the pain pump––and then released me. We went to our friends' again in case something went wrong, but nothing did, so we headed home the next morning.

Maybe it was the pain pump. The next few days went well. I walked, slept, walked, watched television, slept, put in a DVD, and walked. When the pain pump bag emptied after several days, Marti as instructed, pulled the IV tube internal feed out of my side. One of her career options had been to be a nurse. She would have done well.

Her choice of career was teaching physical education, based on the simple logic that wearing comfortable shoes and playing all day equaled a great job. This served me well too. On Monday, the school provided her a personal day. On Tuesday, snow closed the school, meaning she could hover around home in case I needed her. Snow continued and closed school again Wednesday, the day of my appointment to remove the catheter. Given the hundred-mile drive, we called to confirm. If we arrived before their early closing at noon, they would see me. Marti drove forty miles per hour, and we made it.

A friend had told me, "I hated the catheter. It was my least favorite part of recovery. When the nurse removed it three weeks later I wanted to kiss her. Freedom!" He had immediate control of urination and never had to wear a diaper or pads.

We arrived at the surgeon's office and medical complex and waited for a cystoscope to determine if any of my plumbing was leaking. All clear. We waited some more and then were shown to a room for the catheter removal. The removal did not hurt, but my body did not seem like my body. When the tube exited, urine kept exiting as well. The nurse, not prepared for so much volume, quickly grabbed a towel to catch the flow. Helpless to stop the stream, I stood staring at the soaked towel.

They showed me how to put on a diaper. It was clear that I would need it. The diaper was for night, and pads most likely would suffice for day. I took on faith their statement that I would gradually regain control. They warned me that if I experienced urination problems, I should come back. Someone unfamiliar with prostate surgery might attempt to insert a catheter and accidentally undo the stitches used to reattach the urethra. That morning I waddled in with a catheter and now early afternoon waddled out with a diaper.

We began the long, slow drive home. Marti concentrated on the interstate, still accumulating snow. I sat, tired and emotionally muddied. What exactly was I feeling? I became as quiet on the inside as I could and asked God what I was feeling. A get-well card I had received from a friend two months earlier came to mind.

Five years prior, she'd experienced breast cancer. On one of my periodic visits, when she was struggling with depression, I mentioned Psalm 69 as one I read when feeling depressed. In her card to me she mentioned I might need that Psalm for myself again. She was right. I was living the first part of the Psalm:

> *Save me, O God!*
> *For the waters have come up to my neck.*
> *I sink in deep mire,*
> *Where there is no foothold;*
> *I have come into deep waters*
> *And the flood sweeps over me.*
> *I am weary with my crying;*
> *My throat is parched.*
> *My eyes grow dim*
> *Waiting for my God.*

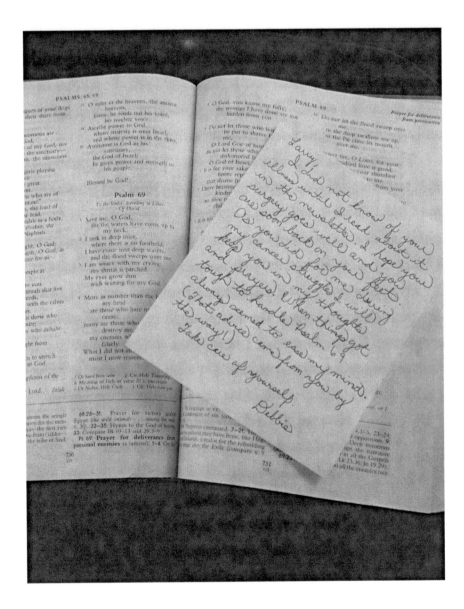

Larry,

I did not know of your illness until I read about it in the newsletter. I hope your surgery goes well and you are soon back on your feet. As you did for me during my cancer struggles I will help you in my thoughts and prayers. When things got tough to handle Psalm 69 always seemed to ease my mind. (That advice came from you by the way!) Take care of yourself

Debbie

I cried. Marti reached over and took my hand. "What's wrong?"

I choked out, "The steps never end."

More deep mire and slick footholds waited back home. That evening, I experienced sharp and long pains in my lower abdomen. The surgeon happened to call: "I have good news. All tissue examined from the surgery was clear. No signs of cancer."

Marti thanked him and added, "He seems to be in a lot of pain."

"Keep taking the pain pills. He will be okay."

Steve the Motorcycle Prostate Man had said, "When my report came back negative indicating no cancer, I pumped my fist and said a loud, 'Thank you God.' I understand my life on earth was loaned to me by God. My loan was still out!"

I did not pump my fist. The pain swallowed the good news of the cancer report.

I slept in the recliner that night, the first of several. Alps slept with me. Actually, Alps slept, and I tried to distract myself from the pain by watching early morning television. Had I pulled out stitches somehow? What was going on? I watched a DVD of Cosby shows during the painless stretches. After the fifth show, I could not bear the pain—or the theme song.

Morning finally came, and I pressed Marti to call the twenty-four hour number the doctor gave us. Someone supposedly stood ready to answer any questions. Not so. A recording said, "Please leave your name and phone number, and a staff member will contact you within twenty-four hours. If you are in extreme pain, go to an emergency room."

If I needed a catheter, an emergency room was not what I wanted. We called again and received the same answer. Another rush of pain came. We went to the emergency room.

Many people ahead of us required care, which turned from annoyance to blessing as the twenty-four hour line called back on our cell phone. The nurse posed several causes: appendicitis, bladder spasm, or origin unknown. We could travel the one hundred miles to see them, or go to our urologist. We heard our family doctor paged at the hospital and decided to call his office. They had an opening in early afternoon, so off we went to him. He immediately ruled out appendicitis, and since our local urologist was in surgery for the day, he called another one for us.

We crossed town, where the urologist checked to see if the bladder was emptying. His sense was the catheter was taken out on the early side (five days), and I was having bladder spasms. Pain pills and medication for the spasms should take care of it. Back home to the recliner and dog I went.

If there was a normal healing process, I was not following it. Whether a reaction to the medication or not eating enough with the medication, I entered a time when not even the dog sat by me. Friday and Saturday, I threw up or dry heaved every two hours. Alps stared at me on the first heave and leapt from the chair, pittered down the hall and hid under the bed.

Finally our family doctor came through again and calmed my system down with an inexpensive over-the-counter drug. I wrote him a thank you note. The dog rejoined me in the chair during the day, and I could sleep in bed at night.

Originally, Marti and I hoped I would feel well enough on this weekend to go with friends for two nights at a bed and breakfast. They came to our house instead. Each of the three male friends witnessed my weariness and said prostate cancer was one more thing on their lists of what not to get.

Sometime later in talking to other men, I found many had side issues in recovery, leading me to think there is no "normal" recovery. The more obvious variables include location and type of cancer, treatment, age, and general physical health. Less obvious variables include each person's reaction to medication, intrusion of treatment, unforeseen complications like size of prostate, and tolerance for pain. Two men can have the same kind of treatment, and one will experience more continence issues or one will achieve ability to erect sooner.

Personality is a crucial factor. How do we respond when events are beyond our control? Do we tend to worry? When vulnerable, do we invite people closer, or keep them at a distance? Do we dwell on the negative, or search quickly for the positive? Are we likely to delay calling for follow-up medical help, or call quickly?

A major difficulty in recovery is the "expectations gap." A patient reviewing literature, listening to medical professionals, or hearing other men's anecdotes, might determine what a normal recovery should be like. Expectations develop as to levels, location, and duration of pain, when one can return to work, urination control, and erectile function. Since few men are normal statistically (and in many other ways!), frustration, anger and depression can fill the gap between what one thought would happen and what actually does happen. This gap is very normal. Other men may not have my complications, but they will have their own aberrations in recovery.

SNAPSHOTS

Mike

Mike strained to look in the toilet after urinating the day after receiving radiation seed implants. Twenty-five of the ninety-three seeds passed. A curious retired engineer, he fished them out of the toilet, stored them away from humans, and took them to his doctor. The doctor's eyes enlarged, and his mouth stood open, pausing for a brain search to find an explanation. Finally his face relaxed, and he said, "It probably happened because the seeds were implanted in a cavity and lost hold, so I do not think there is a problem."

Mike accepted the answer in the moment, but as he waited for his next PSA reading, his anxiety grew. "Are enough seeds left to eradicate the cancer?" he wondered.

Harold

Harold encountered the great misfortune of bad news after his open radical prostatectomy. The cancer had escaped the prostate and attached to the rectum; therefore, the cancer could not be totally removed. Frustration occurred as he received conflicting opinions on the next best course for treatment. He hoped for a clear-cut solution, but instead was forced to sort through options in a short period of time. Urgency required a quick decision.

Not usually one to second-guess, he does second-guess this particular choice of radiation as his treatment after surgery. The radiation also failed to eradicate the cancer and created an additional complication of scar tissue affecting the bladder and urination. Urine leaked into internal cavities, causing infections.

Seeking help for the ongoing urinary infections and blockages, Harold's impression was that each doctor recommended the treatment of his specialty. A doctor not familiar with other treatment options was reluctant to recommend one, even though more fitting for Harold's case. One nurse, out of earshot of the doctor, suggested to Harold he find another doctor with a different approach.

He shifted from trusting doctors to fix his problem, to realizing it is still a "practice" of medicine, and that he needed to manage his own care for his own benefit.

This approach proved effective when his cancer reappeared six years later. He traveled great distances to get the best advice and treatment. He now summarizes his approach to medical care as: Be careful; listen well; seek independent opinions.

Kurt

Kurt's diagnosis occurred in December 2005 at the age of fifty-six. Disturbed, because his father had died horribly of cancer, Kurt wanted to act quickly and thoroughly to remove it. He elected radical prostatectomy surgery via robot. The surgery itself went well, but Kurt experienced a rare side effect caused by his body position on the operating table and his narrow pelvis. Painful neuropathy developed in his legs due to a damaged femoral nerve.

The day after surgery when a nurse wanted him to walk, he complained his legs were hurting and not working. The nurse persisted, and when he stood to walk he collapsed. Pain took over.

Although sent home with medication, the pain only worsened. Medication was changed and changed, but no relief came. His wife, struggling with multiple sclerosis, valiantly tried caring for him, but her own condition deteriorated. Friends from church responded wonderfully and with grace, especially one woman who while changing Kurt's catheter bag was sprayed with urine. Epic constipation set in. Sleep disappeared.

A measure of relief came on the treadmill. If he could bear the pain of walking long enough, his legs would go numb, and the pain subsided for a few hours. He ended up taking a leave from work for a year. Friends from church kept them on their financial feet.

DISCUSSION QUESTIONS

1. When were the low points physically, emotionally, and spiritually?

2. What have been the difficult subjects to talk about?

3. What has changed about your relationship with your partner? Emotionally? Patterns of communication? Physically?

4. As a caregiver, what was it like watching someone you love suffer?

5. As a caregiver, what sustained you? What was not helpful?

6. As a care receiver, what was most helpful to you during this time?

7. Did you have any surprises in recovery?

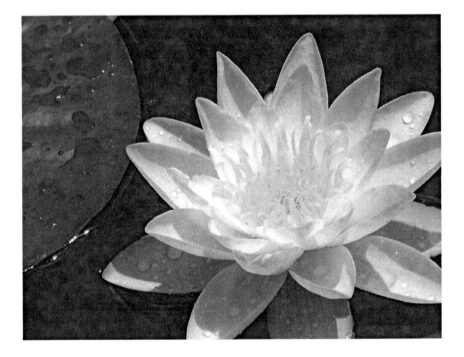

Chapter 5

HOPE

My body settled down. Hope took root. My next painful reaction was to daytime television. Going back to work seemed better than another episode of *Divorce Court* or *Jerry Springer*, so I returned a mere two and a half weeks after surgery.

I wore pads to catch urine leakage, but control was improving. The Kegle exercises of tensing the pelvic and sphincter muscles prior to and post-surgery seemed to be working. Reminders of my tenuous situation still came. One cold afternoon a month into recovery, I walked with a friend. After only forty minutes, urine had filled the pad and saturated the front of my pants. Luckily, a change of clothes lay in the trunk of my car. Six weeks after surgery, I attended a spring training baseball game in Florida and saw wetness darkening the front of my shorts. No one seemed to notice except me. I just stayed seated throughout the game.

At three months, the surgeon told me to stop wearing any pads, so my system would not grow dependent. Pad-free! The occasional spotting on my underwear from forgetting to tense the pelvic and sphincter muscles during sneezes, coughs, or awkward sitting positions was worth it. My investment in Kegle exercises paid dividends.

I was very, very curious about the nerves controlling erection. That curiosity was mixed initially with fear, as I had a catheter in place. What if I accidentally erected? My image was of meat on a kabob, sliding up and down. Marti sexually teased me a few days after surgery, and I cringed, then jerked away in horror.

But one of the first nights home I awoke with a slight erection. My penis was working! The catheter was not a hindrance. Three weeks after the surgery and two weeks after the catheter removal, Marti and I tried to see how big my penis would get. The growth was small but, with the help of KY jelly, the orgasm big. A holy moment!

The next day I was with a group of pastors. The leader asked, "Any big joys or concerns to share with the group?" I smiled.

SNAPSHOTS

Kurt

Kurt found all his familiar ways of connecting to God through prayer and singing severed. A combination of a narrow pelvis and his body position for robotic surgery had produced a damaged femoral nerve. The result was excruciating neuropathy in his legs. For many months his prayer was reduced to, "Help! Help!" No songs flowed from his lips.

With no spirit to sing, he turned to others for help. He started listening to Fernando Ortega's music. Over and over, for hours and hours, Ortega's hymns became Kurt's hymns, giving word, melody, harmony, and rhythm where there had been only despair.

Late one night he phoned a friend who also knew long-term pain. Shot as a youth, he was still in chronic pain. Immediately the friend came to sit with him, and after a time covered him with a prayer: "Dear Lord, sustain my friend Kurt with your grace for however long this healing takes."

What struck Kurt so profoundly was the simple gift of his friend's presence in the midst of pain, and a prayer that did not claim healing or insinuate in any way that Kurt's lack of faith or sin was blocking God's healing. The prayer simply acknowledged

Kurt's long suffering and God's ability to be there, just as his friend was.

Kurt also started to appreciate his wife's steadfastness through the shared ordeal. Her constant friendship was God in the flesh, a hope that sometimes came through humor. They both talked to his penis to encourage erections. Finally, at ten months and two weeks a full erection occurred. More hope!

Their lovemaking changed. Each of them now needs time to get into the mood, he with his slow erection and she with sensory depletion due to the MS. They make a date for lovemaking, marking the calendar with a smiley face. When the date comes, candles, romantic movies, or dancing deepens the intimacy. Reading books on sexual techniques together has led to experimentation with vibrators and oral sex. He does not want their old sex life back. Neither does she. The new one is richer and more loving.

Steve

Steve, the Prostate Motorcycle Man, adopted early in life a sense of gratitude. Gratitude was, in fact, the foundation of his recovery. He was simply grateful to be alive and as free of prostate cancer as one can hope after surgery.

Prior to his open radical prostatectomy, he had already noticed a decline in erection strength, so he sees the further decline from surgery as merely an acceleration of the aging process. He and his wife cuddle and engage in oral sex more for their intimacy. Their relationship is based on more than the rise and fall of the penis.

Russell

Russell, when diagnosed, opted for one year of hormone treatment and then active surveillance. He changed his diet, adding more fruits and vegetables and subtracting red meat. A urologist specializing in analyzing each person's situation and designing a course of action also put him on a vitamin regimen. One of the big changes he made was around work.

Believing that stress contributes to cancer, he took a hard look at his work, or as he calls it, his "false god." To do his work well, which he did, he thrived on being the star salesman, the perennial award winner, the top seller, the aggressive go-getter, the one whom a client wanted to represent their product, the one who made the most money.

He first identified which area in his job contributed the most stress. These were the clients who compelled him to change his basic nature to please. He began carefully picking his clients. Next, he lowered the number of hours he worked. Gradually, he retired completely. He misses being in charge, respected, and recognized. But when the temptation comes to get back into his field, he asks himself, "What's really important?"

For him quality of life is important. He and his wife started living in Florida where each day is a "complete wonder" of joy. Tennis, followed by schmoozing with the boys, leads to lunch and puttering with his old Corvette. Children, especially grandchildren, receive special attention.

He recalled a recent night with his small grandson. "As he sat on my lap, and we read a book, he wrapped his tiny hand around my finger. I did not want the story to end. I did not want that magic moment of love and trust to end. My voice faltered as I turned the last page. He was so unaware of the gift he was giving me."

Russell could barely tell this story to me for the tears escaping his concealing eyelids.

In Florida, Russell goes to a Wellness Community support group for men with a variety of cancers. Several men shared how cancer became one of the best things to happen to them, as they began to shift priorities and make decisions based on what they held most precious, usually family. Russell experienced himself in their sharing. Cancer had been a gift to him. The last nine years with the disease clarified his values and deepened relationships. Life became more precious. If the cancer does spread and death comes, at this moment he can say he has no regrets about his decision to practice what he calls active surveillance.

With phrases like " inner voice," "complete wonder," and "false god," you might expect Russell to be practicing a faith. He is not. He does not feel connected to God. He does practice love more than ever and is grateful for each day, which in some religious traditions is connection with God. God is bigger than the definitions we assign.

Harold

Since Harold's cancer lay outside the prostate, he is glad just to be alive and enjoying life in small ways. He is sixteen years past his diagnosis at age forty-eight. He loves to garden, turning his back yard into a peaceful paradise. Planting lettuce each spring harbors hope. If he sits out on his deck, it is not long until the neighbor boy comes over for the customary lemonade. Then they play ball.

During initial consultations about the cancer, Harold was told he would still have sexual function. Due to the cancer being outside the prostate and complications with his treatments, Harold's nerves controlling erection were destroyed. Initially he still had an orgasm. He tried two kinds of prostheses, but one did not work well, and the second burst, causing infections. Eventually his testicles were removed. Due to incontinence, he does not feel very sexy.

His sexual expressions are now hugging, kissing, and cuddling. He misses the "us" part that sexual intercourse and orgasm bring to intimacy. Yet he still feels like a man and that his core personhood is intact. While struggling to come to terms with his sexual mechanical problem, he saw the movie *Little Big Man*. One of the characters is missing a new appendage with each appearance, yet is still enthusiastic. No matter how many arms or legs he loses, he still remains upbeat. So does Harold. He and his wife continue to practice physical closeness through hugging, kissing, cuddling, and going to an occasional bed and breakfast.

Ruth

One spouse, Ruth, exclaimed their sex life was good before surgery––but after surgery, it is great. She always needed more time to be aroused, and now they both need time. One game they play is to take turns pleasing each other. Whoever's turn it is to receive, gets to request the nature of touching. The giver gives without any expectations for self. No intercourse is involved. The next time they switch roles. They've found new hot spots after twenty-five years of marriage.

Doug

When first hearing of his cancer, Doug sighed deeply, "Why me, Lord?" The cancer arrived on top of his wife's chronic health difficulties and their son's alcohol addiction. Sitting in despondency, he remembered the core wisdom of Al-anon in his son's addiction. "I didn't cause it; I can't cure it; I can't control it; I can cope with it." Short-term coping involved research and selection of treatment and open communication with his wife. Long-term coping relied on longtime disciplines of personal devotions with God and participation in a small support group from church. Hope edged its way into the many questions and doubts. And there are doubts, like if the radiation seeds are really doing their job.

Tim

Tim slipped into major depression when an erection did not occur after surgery. He got drunk for the first time in his life. He toyed with ways he could kill himself. His wife suggested counseling, but that did not seem to help. Then he went to a prostate cancer support group, and the connection with other men let him know he was not alone, and gave him practical steps to work on erectile dysfunction.

DISCUSSION QUESTIONS

1. What were the signs of hope for you physically, particularly in regard to urination and erections?
2. What were the emotional highs?
3. What was nourishing you spiritually?
4. How did you celebrate new achievements?
5. Who were the people who were most helpful to be around?
6. What new learnings have you and your partner discovered in lovemaking?

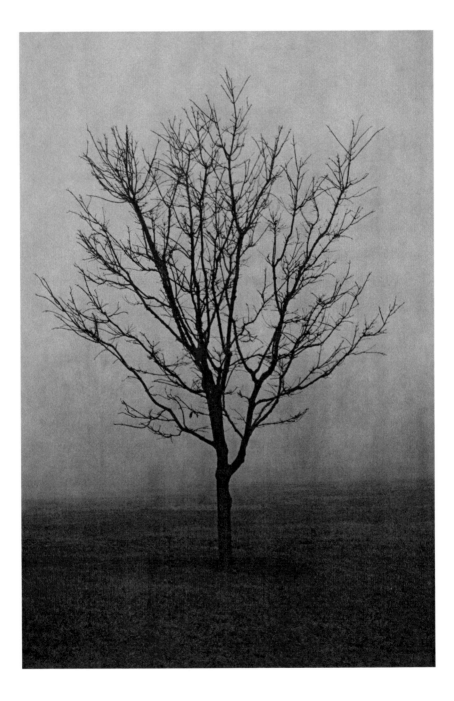

CHAPTER 6

LOSS

Before cancer, I loved starting my day with jogging, then eating breakfast while reading the newspaper, then showering, and then sitting in the recliner to pray. I gradually returned to the routine, except the jogging was slower, and the prayer quickly slid into sleep. Reading at night resulted in the same. I kept reading bits of Scripture and writing in a journal, but as the days of spring arrived, my spirit lagged behind the calendar.

Looking back, several things occurred. My workload increased as we lost some key staff members. I contracted a urinary tract infection the week before Easter, my busiest week of the year. And I entered erectile dysfunction therapy, also known as my pump-pill-and-prick season.

I entered this whole new world hopefully, guided by a nurse specializing in erectile dysfunction. The first aid was a pump. Twice a day I greased the edge of the pump, like putting oil on an oil filter gasket to make a seal, and then put the long pump cylinder over my penis and flat against the surrounding tissue. It is critical to leave one's testicles outside the cylinder! Slowly pressing down on a lever creates a vacuum. Slow is also critical. The vacuum brings blood into the penis. My new early morning routine consisted of push-ups, crunches, jogging, and penis pumping.

Provided with the pump were semi-elastic rings. These slipped over the pumped-up penis, thereby keeping blood inside and making intercourse possible. I don't know if it was those warnings I'd heard as a child not to leave a rubber band too long and too tight around my finger, or the finger would lose blood, turn black, and fall off––or the memory of snapping a rubber band and the sharp pain. Whatever it was, I chose just to use the pump for exercise.

The second P was a pill. These pills had become infamous on television commercials for their warning of a four-hour erection. I was hoping for a few minutes. Depending on the brand, erections could begin anywhere from one half-hour after taking the pill and be effective up to twenty-four hours later. The pill, plus fondling, equaled erection. Each person reacts to the drug in a different way. I developed most of the side effects listed: face flushing, flu-like symptoms, and headaches. Creating a headache in order to make love became a deterrent, but was well worth the effort! Planning replaced spontaneity, but it too was well worth the effort!

The third P was prick. I was trained to give myself an injection in my penis that resulted in an erection within ten minutes. The procedure involved cleansing the injection site with alcohol, twisting the penis so the needle would not puncture the nerves running along the top of it, and selecting a spot that did not have many veins.

Perhaps if I had drunk the alcohol, my courage would have overcome my fears. I passed the first test of injecting myself in front of the therapist, though I did drop the needle and had to start over. I successfully accomplished about six shots on my own. There are reasons I did not become a doctor, and administering shots is one of them. Though there was very little pain with injection, the whole psychological barrier to giving myself a shot in the penis only grew. I had a thirty-second window to give myself the shot, or my hand started to shake. Shaking hands miss the target. Or bend needles. Which results in, "I'm too stressed out and nervous from my shot tonight; can we wait for another romantic moment?"

One prostate cancer friend did well with the shot. He was a biology teacher. Maybe years of dissection carried crossover skills. I heard many months later from a urologist at a gathering sponsored by the Urology Group of Cincinnati that about half of the men trying injections quit within a year. The upside for those who inject is a seventy-five to eighty-five percent success rate of erection suitable for penetration.

Several peculiar aspects of sexual recovery surfaced for me. One was the combination of urinary control and sexual activity. Several times I peed on Marti as my erection grew. I apologized.

She chuckled. We continued. To begin lovemaking, standing up helped blood flow to the penis. Clumsily, we experimented with the best moment to head for bed before the erection whimpered out. Penetration on my part was soft. Over the months, what worked best for us was mutual caressing of our private areas. I still pump. I no longer prick. When I take a pill, penetration can happen. We are finding our way to mutual pleasure.

By the end of May, I was exhausted. Looking back, I should have taken more time off work. I fell asleep if I sat in a comfortable chair. I went to bed early. I angered more quickly. I cried more readily. Once I watched a poorly produced film with friends. A person was dying of an illness in a trite way, and they were laughing. I wept. Death was no longer a distant image on the screen for me.

Another time I was playing cards with my folks, and my mom mentioned that some of her friends who go to my church said I really looked tired. I teared up. I thought I was portraying good energy, but apparently I was deceiving myself. Others saw me clearly in ways that I did not want to see myself.

That night I dreamed. I was playing basketball, and every pass that came my way went bounding past me, just beyond my reach. Each rebound ricocheted to another player who stretched slightly higher. My tiredness weighed me down, preventing me from reaching or jumping up. I woke. The dream was my life. My energy, my emotions, and even my penis could not get up like they used to.

I shared the tired part with my personnel committee, and they offered me a month off. I postponed accepting their offer until after my summer vacation, to see if that would refresh me. My vacation goals were simple that year: rest and exercise. The rest evaporated as soon as I returned to work. I felt dropped by God. No energy, no vision, no patience. I started to count my losses: loss of invincibility; loss of complete urine control; loss of sex as I had known it; loss of energy for work.

My calendar had no room for cancer.

I went for my six-month checkup with the surgeon and asked, "I seem to be so low on energy and enthusiasm; could it be depression?"

"No. Men only get depressed the first week after surgery."

Not true, I thought.

As I discovered a year later while doing research for this writing, my intuition was correct. Depression is often part of recovery. A man told the healthlink line of the University of Wisconsin Medical School, "I just had surgery for prostate cancer. My doctor tells me the operation was successful, and all the cancerous tissue was removed. There was also no evidence the disease has spread. Despite all the good news——why am I still feeling down in the dumps?"

Russel G. Robertson, M.D. responded, "Keep in mind that almost any form of surgery can adversely affect one's notion of health and invincibility. Signs of depression include: excessive fatigue, sleeplessness, too much sleep, crying episodes, a significant increase or decrease in appetite, a loss of ambition or motivation, and in some cases, self-destructive thoughts. The result may be an episode of depression that can be brief or long-lasting. For some, just recognizing there may be a cause-and-effect relationship is liberating enough to offer hope for eventual resolution without intervention. For others, especially if the symptoms worsen or show no sign of relenting after a few weeks, consultation with your doctor is definitely in order."

Most often it is the partner who sees the signs of depression, not the man. John Greden, M.D. and director of the Michigan University Depression Center writes, "Depression remains the 'under' disease: under-diagnosed, under-discussed, and under-treated for everyone, but especially for men. Men tend to focus on physical rather than emotional ailments––for example, fatigue, physical pain, and sleep problems."

A friend spotted the symptoms in her husband. She wanted to yell, "William, get off your butt and do something!" He was taking another midday nap. There was wood to be cut to heat them through winter and lawn to mow on their fifty acres. He'd never napped before, much less the current hour or two. Plus, he was cranky. He even scheduled an appointment with their pastor to read a list of everything the pastor was doing wrong. In a class William was auditing, he accidentally skipped a question on a homework assignment and got an A- instead of an A+. He grumbled all day about his stupidity.

What his wife did say was, "At your next visit, why don't you tell your doctor you don't have any energy?"

At his six-month follow-up, he shared with the intake nurse, "I'm not my old self energy-wise. I keep dragging and needing naps. My wife says I'm more short-tempered than usual."

"That's not surprising," she responded, "your body is still healing, and will be for another year or two. Most men get depressed over what they think is a slow return of continence and potency. I'm glad you said something. Most men seldom say anything, thinking it is a sign of weakness. I recommend you go to your family doctor and talk to him about what you are experiencing. He might put you on some medication that will take an edge off your depression."

That is exactly what happened. His family doctor rarely gave out prescriptions, but he concurred immediately. It took four weeks, just as the doctor had said, for the pill to make a difference. But that difference improved his mental state.

His wife no longer is tempted to tell him, "Get off your butt!"

Three months after my surgeon told me depression occurred only the first week after surgery, I went to a career-counseling center for clergy and underwent a battery of psychological and interest tests. They were not surprised I felt depressed. All my scores indicated I was! I felt both relief and sadness. Relief in having a name for what I felt, but sadness in my distress. What to do? What I did not know was that in the depression something new was coming to life. The unknown "new" just needed room.

SNAPSHOTS

Joe

Joe should be dead. Six times. Four times in the military, and twice with illness. There are days he wishes he were dead, but God keeps him from pulling the trigger.

He chose radiation for treatment. One result was the end of his sex life with his wife of fifty-one years, his one true love. The cancer stayed in remission for four years and then came back. Hormone therapy ensued, which contained the spread for several years. Meanwhile he was diagnosed with Parkinson's. His wife died on her birthday. A daughter with power-of-attorney drained his finances, feeding a drug addiction. She died on Christmas Day. When the cancer spread over his urethra, his testes were removed. Now he urinates two to seven times a night.

Incredulous, I asked him, "What helps you keep going on?"

"I talk myself out of 'poor me.' I have long, intense conversations with God, letting God filter the anger and disappointment. Then I focus on what God has given me: a roof, plenty of food, children, and grandchildren."

He limps along as best he can, carting both tragedy and blessings, his faith resolute. The afterlife glows ahead of him, and he thinks his actions on this side of death determine his eternity. So he and God continue to keep his finger off the trigger of his service revolver.

DISCUSSION QUESTIONS

1. When were your low moments in recovery?
2. What helped or hindered you during these difficult times?
3. Has your partner seen any signs of depression, such as irritability, tiredness, loss of joy, or loss of sleep?
4. What losses would you name as having experienced through this?
5. What pleasures you sexually besides intercourse?
6. What helps you to stay emotionally intimate with your partner?

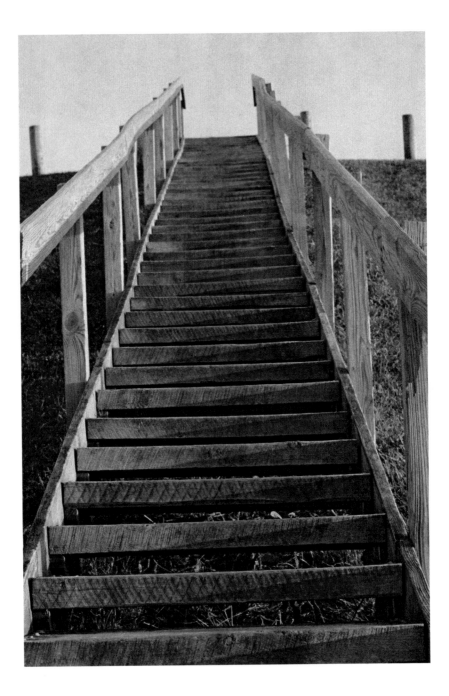

Chapter 7

ROOM

For no particular reason, I chose to read one Psalm each day for my daily devotional. The fourth day Psalm 4:1 brought my struggle into focus. My paraphrase is, "Out of my distress I called upon the Lord, and the Lord gave me room."

Room. Space. Enlarge. All words associated with the Hebrew word for salvation.

To deliver, to be broad, to become spacious, to enlarge. Just the opposite of being compressed, confined, or constrained in some sense. Depression is a form of being pressed down, compressed. One's hope diminishes under its weight.

My depression was mild by clinical standards, but its weight plagued me. I felt stuck, unable to move beyond my present despondency.

Some therapists call depression frozen anger, stemming from sadness, hurt, or disappointment that gets stuck within us. Others speak of depression as a sign of an old paradigm shifting and a new understanding of life coming, a grief over losing the old. The depression may be related to a temporary situation in one's life, such as illness or a difficult situation at work. Chemical imbalance, either temporary or permanent, can bring changes in mood. I was searching for room, a new space, a saving from my stuckness.

Thankfully, I found out I was not alone. One friend asked me how I was I doing, and I shared with her my tiredness and depression. She nodded knowingly. Two years earlier, she had received a kidney transplant and was sailing through recovery, when the wind changed direction, and her energy fluttered to a stop. She contacted her doctor, and he gently said, "We have been waiting for this. You lost a major part of your body. Your body, which you have counted on all these years, has let you down by getting gravely ill. Depression is natural. It is part of the recovery."

I told her story and my story together in a sermon, and a woman from my congregation came up to me afterward and spoke about her depression with breast cancer. Her doctor told her that during her long struggle for recovery she'd used up the antidepressant chemicals in her body and needed to have them replaced chemically. The medication helped her to engage life with more energy.

Another friend, ten years on the other side of her cancer, shared her journey with depression. "You cannot know when the depression will end. You cannot will it to end. You may never get your energy back to the level you once enjoyed. But you can do things to help: go to therapy, make different decisions about career, use alternative forms of healing, let people love and support you. Depression leaves in its own time."

Mine was a lonely place. These friends entered with understanding and compassion. Misery is blessed by company.

One day a lady, whose husband had died a couple of years earlier, stopped by the church. She was struggling with what to do with her life. She did not need to work, but she did need purpose and worthwhile activity. Much of her life had centered on her children, now grown, and her husband, now gone.

Her wrestling touched my own turbulence, and I reflected back, "I'm feeling some guilt. I am fortunate. My cancer was detected early, and most likely my life expectancy is not shortened, so it seems I should be happy. It seems I should be clear on what to do with this gift of life. But I'm not happy, and I don't have a clear vision of what to do with the rest of my life. I am depressed and cannot see beyond the depression. Usually I have a vision and a plan for what is next. I don't right now. I'm just waiting. Hoping. What do I want to do with the rest of my life? How would God like to use me?"

Waiting is hard, whether waiting to hear a biopsy report, deciding on treatment or discerning what is next in life. A practice for me over the years is to have a spiritual director or companion, someone with whom I can share what I am experiencing in life and look for God's movement.

During this time of depression, my spiritual director, who was also a therapist, kept inviting me to let the depression run its course and open the future on its own time schedule. The battery of tests I took at the career center said my depression was mild, and I was not a danger to others or myself.

Medication was an option, but my depression seemed situational around the experience of cancer and my coming to an end of serving my church of fourteen years and our completion of a building addition. Not only did I suffer from lack of personal vision, I lacked energy for the congregation's future vision. They needed more from my leadership.

One day I mused with my spiritual director on my "stuckness." One of the personality types on the Meirs-Briggs Personality inventory is to be orderly and punctual, to complete assignments on time, and to have a plan. The letter "J" denotes this trait. I am a strong "J." He suggested letting the opposite trait out, which includes spontaneity, keeping options open, and dreaming of possibilities. The letter "P" denotes this trait. I mused, "So its time to let my Pee out?" How fitting. I started to dream.

At about this time, two books came into my life. A good friend who'd listened well throughout the whole ordeal sent Parker Palmer's book, *Let Your Life Speak*. Palmer suffered bouts of severe depression and spoke of one of his turning points. A friend pointed out that he could fight the depression or let it be a friend, a friend who pushed him down into the gentle hands of God, who would be faithful in holding him.

I closed the book and invited God to use the depression to press me down into caring hands for re-forming. A measure of peace came. I began to move from struggling––to listening to what I was experiencing and what might be forming.

The second book arrived unsolicited in the mail at my office. I usually throw those out after a casual glance at the titles. Most of them have been predictions of dates when Jesus was coming again, all which have since come and gone.

The Dream Manager, written by business consultant Matthew Kelly, told the parable of a custodial service company that was experiencing high employee turnover. The company tried a totally new approach to retain its employees. They hired a Dream Maker. The Dream Maker listened to employees and helped put into words their personal dreams and plans to aid their birth.

Dreams, such as buying a home or having reliable transportation, slowly became reality. Employees obviously benefited, but so did the company. Current employees stayed longer, because they felt the company cared about their dreams, and the pool of applicants increased, as others wanted to work in a place where dreams came true.

The timing was right for me. I let my "P" out. I wrote a list of dreams. My room expanded.

SNAPSHOTS

Doug

Though he feels his afterlife is covered in his relationship with Christ, the diagnosis of cancer triggered earthly changes for Doug. He started a widow's file with important financial and end-of-life papers, finished the decade long do-it-yourself basement remodeling by hiring a professional, and reevaluated his activities as to their significance. Currently he works with Habitat for Humanity, prepares tax returns for elders in AARP, and performs random acts of kindness through his church. Does he want to change or add to any of his activities?

Mike

Mental state is his strong suit. When Mike began thinking retirement twenty years ago, he wanted to make sure he had plenty to do. Raising his three children, he always enjoyed participating in hobbies with them, from model-powered airplanes to fossil hunting to a model custom-designed car. Given his passion for hobbies, the first eight years of retirement he researched and wrote about *Favorite Hobbies and Pastimes*, publishing a book of three hundred pages.

Now in his eighties and with a recent radical prostatectomy, he uses the same mental framework that served him well when he retired. Mike teaches a senior citizen class for twenty-five men on model boats, airplanes and cars. He does research each week to prepare, and tracks down the men who miss a couple weeks in a row.

By keeping his mind active and his hands busy, he keeps his mind on what he has, rather than on what he has lost. He is looking past his eighties toward his nineties.

SUPPORT GROUP

One day in a small group setting in our Cancer Wellness Community, I asked if anyone had "lost" something in the cancer experience that they were happy to lose. The answers were intriguing. One woman lost her shyness and found her voice, now speaking out on injustices. A man is no longer interested in watching sports on television and instead spends more time with his grandchildren. Another man, who was always asking God, "Why?" in a cynical way about all of life's circumstances, is more contented to live with the questions. A woman, who was always the caregiver of others, now extends more care to herself. Loss makes room for the new.

DISCUSSION QUESTIONS

1. What gifts have you experienced through cancer?
2. How is your life different now?
3. Draw a timeline of your cancer experience. Place painful or negative experiences below the line and joyful and positive experiences above the line. What do you observe?
4. Are there things you have "lost" in the cancer experience for which you are grateful?
5. What are your dreams for the future? What would you like to do sooner rather than later? What is on your "bucket list" of things to do before you die?

Chapter 8

HEAR

During my recovery, my quiet time with God in the recliner each morning usually resulted in a nap. Reading long passages of Scripture or challenging books resulted in a nap. These connections severed, I depended more on my Gratitude and Dear Lord journals for my fragile link to God. When I wrote I stayed awake. I journaled a list of dreams and explored them on paper for a few days. A particular one kept coming to the forefront, one that I tried to do off and on over the years, with more off than on: Write.

Parts of my job involve writing or verbal forms of creative expression. I write a monthly newsletter to the congregation. A weekly sermon, though unwritten, gives me a chance to research, observe life, and make connections with God. I longed to do more. Several years before, I tried writing on my day off but soon found a day off needed to be a day off. Writing took energy. Was now the time to write? Was the experience of cancer creating room for something new?

Parker Palmer gave encouragement again. He underscored that there are times in our lives when we need to love ourselves in order to love others. Seldom is an act of self-love a selfish endeavor.

Two things became clear to me. I no longer had the vision or energy to serve my present church. And presently, I did not have the energy, desire, or vision to lead a different church.

In talking to one of our denominational leaders, a third option developed, growing over time into the one we selected. I could leave my present church and take a year's sabbatical, with the denomination paying for our hospitalization plan and pension contribution. If we left the church, we also needed to leave the church-owned house, but Marti's teaching salary and our savings easily covered all anticipated expenses.

The idea of a sabbatical fit my need for room, space, enlargement, and salvation. I imagined my life as a field in the ancient Hebrew tradition, left in the seventh year to be fallow and replenish. The field was wide and expansive. What new experiences and opportunities lay dormant, waiting for their opportunity for life above ground? I tingled in wonderment.

I tested my intentions with family, friends, and a few church leaders. The leaders were disappointed that I would leave, but thought it sounded best for me. Family and friends supported the idea. When I finally committed to the sabbatical with my denominational leaders, I danced in the parking lot.

On the back page of my journal I began a list of writing projects. On the second to last page I began a list of places I wanted to visit. Several were of a spiritual nature, places where pilgrims had gone over the centuries: the Camino Pilgrimage across the northern top of Spain, the Franciscan Trail in Italy, and the town of Crestone, Colorado. Making the list, I suddenly realized I was already on a long, sacred journey. Whether I traveled geographically or not, the last two years with cancer had led me deeper and deeper into unknown terrain in search for the sacred. I was on a pilgrimage. I was a pilgrim.

As I spent time in quiet, recording thoughts in my journal, and shared my searching with others, clarity began to emerge. I needed time to replenish my body, mind, and spirit. I wanted to write, particularly about the emotional, spiritual, and sexual aspects of prostate cancer recovery.

Leaving our church family of fourteen years was freeing and sad. Love flowed both ways. I found incredible meaning and joy in being a representative of God's presence in people's hurts and joys. I did not dance when Marti and I left. We mourned. I also felt wonderfully drawn to something new.

There were many beautiful acts of saying goodbye. One night, our worship-planning group had a person sit in a chair as proxy for the new pastor. We laid hands on her head and prayed for the pastor who was yet to come. Then they had me sit in the chair. Laying hands on my head and shoulders, they gave thanks for my ministry. They anointed my writing hand with oil for the sabbatical year ahead.

Four-year old Sam told his Sunday school teacher, "Larry is leaving, and he is changing his name."

She answered, "Yes, Larry is leaving, but he will still be Larry."

"No," he said with conviction. "His name is Arthur."

"Honey, I'm sure he will still be Larry."

"My mom said, he will be Arthur."

Finally the teacher got it! "You are right! He is going to be an author!"

Sam made his mom take him shopping and then come to my office with his goodbye gift. I opened the bag, and there was a notebook, pen, and colored markers. On my last Sunday I shared a children's story, illustrated with his markers. I use his pen now to write in my journal.

I am now on sabbatical. Marti and I spent last summer traveling to photographic seminars for her and a writing workshop for me. Our children are spread across the Midwest, and we stayed with each of them. We made it to Crestone, Colorado, home to twenty-five different religious expressions and stayed in a monastery for three nights. I exercise an hour each day and attend a variety of support groups at our local Wellness Community. We are changing our diets, and we bought a sex manual.

I am less irritable, but have managed to pick a few fights with my wife. I still feel experiences deeply, but no longer feel on the edge of my emotions all the time. I noticed one Sunday in worship that I was experiencing what the Psalmist proclaimed, "I was glad when they said unto me, let us go into the House of the Lord." Joy felt good.

One night I went to a function sponsored by our local urology group on incontinence and erectile dysfunction. One hundred men and a few partners attended. We were introduced to the newest gadgets and improvements. As I looked around the room, I saddened. When I went home I sat next to Marti on the couch as she watched television. She asked, "How was it?"

Once again I felt tears forming as I shared, "Not so good."

She turned off the television and looked at me. I continued, "I was the youngest one there."

I pity-partied for a day or so and then went on with living. At least the pity parties are less intense and frequent than before.

I do write, sometimes enthusiastically, sometimes ploddingly. Interviewing men and their partners about prostate cancer has been a sacred privilege. As men share, they make new connections about the meaning of cancer in their lives. So do I. We get teary-eyed together.

One year ago on my birthday I was depressed. Two years ago I had a catheter inserted and a diagnosis of prostate cancer. This year I celebrated my fifty-fifth birthday with fifty-five push-ups, fifty-five sit-ups and fifty-five minutes of jogging.

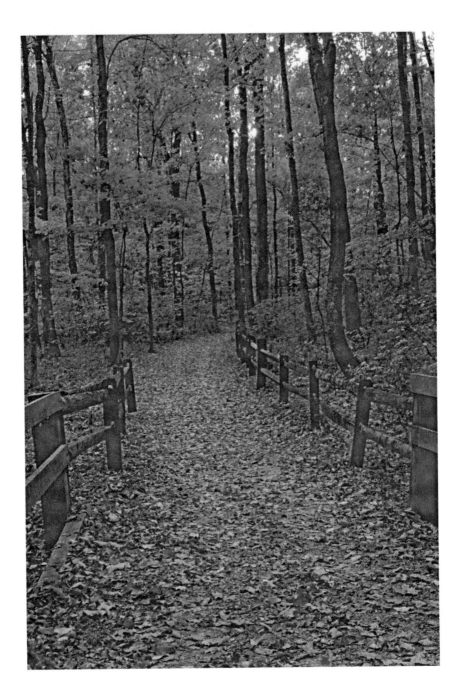

On the run through the gorge in the park, I was nearing the fifty-five minute mark and raised my arms in triumph. Raising my arms also raised my head, and I missed seeing a root on the trail. Down I went. But up I bounced. So life goes.

Looking toward my two-year anniversary of surgery, I continue the pilgrimage, the sacred journey with cancer as an act of devotion to God. I did not know in the fall of 2006 that I was beginning a pilgrimage into cancer. But I was. Twenty-five years ago I did not know I would share my grandfather's journey. But I did. And through all the fear, love, pain, hope, and loss, I am extremely grateful for the room I have been given to hear God and be open to a new life. Cancer is a long, sacred journey. It is my journey, and thankfully, I am not alone. We are not alone.

DISCUSSION QUESTIONS

1. In what ways has your experience with cancer been a sacred pilgrimage?
2. As you move farther away from diagnosis and treatment, how have your feelings changed?
3. What lifestyle changes have you made or do you plan to make?
4. Whom would you like to thank for being there with you on your journey?
5. How will you go about thanking them?

RESOURCES FOR THE PILGRIMAGE

Resources we turn to often have a cumulative rather than dramatic impact. Over time they enhance our wholeness of mind, body, and spirit.

THOSE AROUND US

God

Family and friends

Faith communities

Local prostate cancer support groups (see www.ustoo.org and www.cancer.org. below)

Local counselors and spiritual directors

BOOKS

A Primer on Prostate Cancer: The Empowered Patient's Guide. Stephen Strum and Donna Pogliano.

Dr. Patrick Walsh's Guide to Surviving Prostate Cancer, Second Edition. Patrick Walsh and Janet Ferrar Worthington.

Dr. Peter Scardino's Prostate Book: The Complete Guide to Overcoming Prostate Cancer, Prostatitis and BPH. Peter Scardino and Judith Kelman.

Intimacy with Impotence: The Couple's Guide to Better Sex after Prostate Disease. Ralph and Barbara Alterowitz.

WEBSITES

www.cancer.org. Man to Man, an organization sponsored by the American Cancer Association, offers programs and support for men and their families coping with the treatment and side effects of prostate cancer. Search for Man to Man on their website. Phone: 1-800-ACS-2345.

www.menstuff.org/resources/resourcefiles/prostate.html. Lists over one hundred links to prostate cancer resources.

www.msnbc.msn.com/id/13154507/ Prostate cancer is a triple whammy for men, threatening incontinence, impotence, and death. MSNBC.com writer Mike Sturkey chronicles his journey from diagnosis through treatment as he learns more about his disease, his options, and himself.

www.pcri.org. Prostate Cancer Research Institute's mission is to improve the quality of men's lives by supporting research and disseminating information that educates and empowers patients, families, and the medical community. Helpline: 1-800-641-PCRI.

www.prostate-cancer-institute.org/index/html. Prostate Cancer Institute offers information for prostate patients and their families. Phone 1-866-469-7733.

www.psa-rising.com. PSA Rising offers news, information, and support for prostate cancer survivors.

www.renewintimacy.org. The Center for Intimacy after cancer therapy.

www.thewellnesscommunity.org. Check for a Wellness Community near you that offers cancer support, education, and hope. They offer a variety of support groups for cancer survivors and their families.

www.ustoo.org Prostate Cancer Education and Support for men with prostate cancer and their families.

ABOUT THE AUTHOR

Larry Kreps was diagnosed with prostate cancer at age 53. Many times as a pastor, huddled with a family in a hospital waiting room, he heard the word "cancer" when a doctor shared with the family the outcome of a biopsy. These experiences did not protect him from the same shock and fear of hearing his own diagnosis: CANCER.

The cancer came toward the end of a four- teen year pastorate at John Wesley United Methodist in Cincinnati, the building of a church addition, the last child leaving home and general tiredness. The cancer capsized his emotional, physical and spiritual well-being. He became depressed. He searched for ways to regain a satisfying sex life with his wife, wandering through a maze of pumps, pills and needle pricks. The love of God that held him up preceding and during surgery seemed to drop him in the midst of recovery.

Worn out, he stepped out of his career and responsibilities for a year's sabbatical. The depression proved to be situational. A new way of relating sexually as a couple delightfully emerged. The sense of God's presence erupted in color on a gorge path in October.

Larry now serves St. Andrew's United Methodist Church in Findlay, Ohio. He actively pursues his "sooner than later list," those things he wants to do with his gift of renewed life. They include hiking down and up the Grand Canyon with his family, playing golf on what use to be the family farm, writing, and his new ministry goal: show up and have fun.

LaVergne, TN USA
18 February 2010
173505LV00002B/1/P